Lean and Green Air Fryer Meat Cookbook

An Innovative Diet Plan to Stay Fit and Healthy

Roxana Sutton

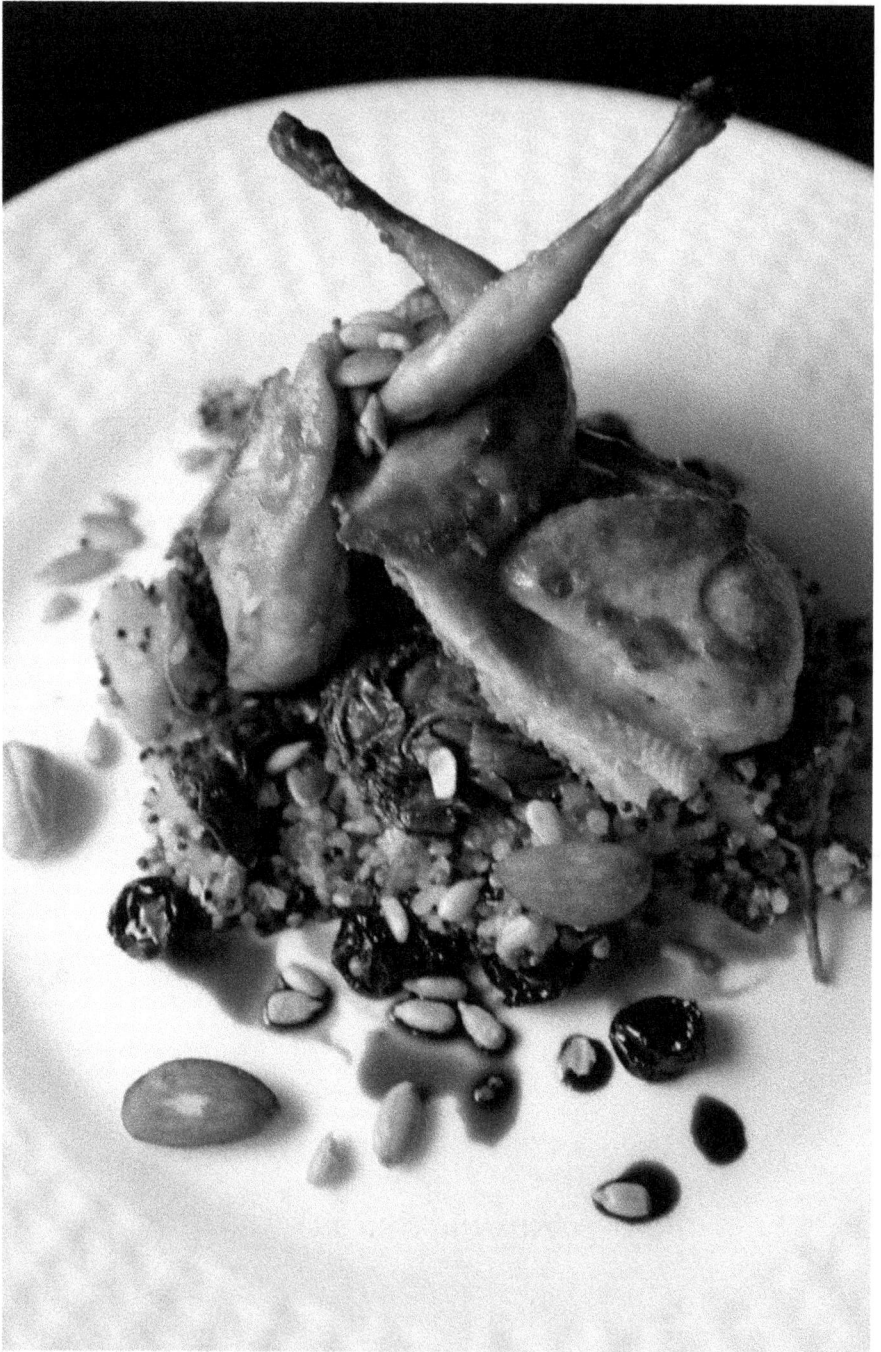

TABLE OF CONTENTS

Air fryer Steak Tips

Prep Time: 5 minutes

Cook Time: 9 minutes

Total Time: 14 minutes

 Servings: 3

Ingredients

- 1.5 lb steak or beef chuck for a cheaper version cut to 3/4 inch cubes
- Air Fryer Steak Marinade
- 1 tsp oil
- 1/4 tsp salt
- 1/2 tsp black pepper, freshly ground
- 1/2 tsp dried garlic powder
- 1/2 tsp dried onion powder
- 1 tsp Montreal Steak Seasoning
- 1/8 tsp cayenne pepper
- Air Fryer Asparagus
- 1 lb Asparagus, tough ends trimmed (could replace with spears of zucchini)
- 1/4 tsp salt
- 1/2 tsp oil (optional)

Instructions

Preheat the air fryer at 400F for about 5 minutes.

Meanwhile, trim the steak of any fat and cut it into cubes. Then, toss with the ingredients for the marinade (oil, salt, black pepper, Montreal seasoning, onion and garlic powder & the cayenne pepper) and massage the spices into the meat to coat evenly. Do this in a ziplock bag for easier cleanup.

Spray the bottom of the air fryer basket with nonstick spray if you have any and spread the prepared meat along the bottom of it. Cook the beef steak tips for about 4-6 minutes and check for doneness.

Toss the asparagus with 1/2 tsp oil and 1/4 tsp salt until evenly coated.

Once the steak bites are browned to your liking, toss them around and move to one side. Add the asparagus to the other side of the air fryer basket and cook for another 3 minutes.

Remove the steak tips and the asparagus to a serving plate and serve while hot.

Nutrition Facts

Calories:526||Fat:34g|SaturatedFat:14g|Cholesterol:138mg|Sodium:703mg|Potassium:913mg|Carbohydrates:6g|Fiber:3g|Sugar:2g|Protein: 49g|Calcium: 52mg|Iron: 7.1mg

Easy Air Fryer Steak Bites

Prep Time: 5 minutes

Cook Time: 9 minutes

Total Time: 14 minutes

Yield: 2-4 servings

Ingredients

- Sirloin Steak Bites or a 1lb. sirloin steak cut into bite-size pieces
- Steak seasoning or salt and pepper
- Olive oil

Instructions

Start by preheating your air fryer to 390° or 400°.

Place the steak bites in a bowl and add about a tablespoon of steak seasoning or season with salt and pepper.

Pour in a tablespoon of olive oil and toss to coat all of the steak bites.

Place the steak bites in a single layer in your air fryer basket and cook for 5 minutes.

Turn the steak bites over and cook for an additional 4 minutes for a medium steak. Cook for an additional 2-3 minutes for medium-well and a couple of minutes less for medium-rare.

Remove from the air fryer and allow them to rest for 5-10 minutes so the meat will retain its juices. Enjoy a salad or with your favorite veggies for lunch or dinner!

Nutritional Value

Calories: 572kcal | Carbohydrates: 1g | Protein: 46g | Fat: 43g | Saturated Fat: 22g | Cholesterol: 168mg

| Sodium: 219mg | Potassium: 606mg | Sugar: 1g | Calcium: 16mg | Iron: 4mg

Air Fryer Steak Bites (With Or Without Potatoes)

Prep Time: 10 mins

Cook Time: 20 mins

Total Time: 30 mins

Servings: 4 Servings

Ingredients

- 1 lb. (454 g) steaks, cut into 1/2" cubes & patted dry
- 1/2 lb. (227 g) potatoes (optional), cut into 1/2" pieces
- 2 tablespoons (30 ml) butter, melted (or oil)
- 1 teaspoon (5 ml) worcestershire sauce
- 1/2 teaspoon (2.5 ml) garlic powder
- Salt, to taste
- Black pepper, to taste
- Minced parsley, garnish
- Melted butter for finishing, optional
- Chili flakes, for finishing, optional

Instructions

Heat a large pot of water to a boil and then add the potatoes. Cook for about 5 minutes, or until nearly tender, and then drain.

Combine the steak cubes and blanched potatoes. Coat with the melted butter and then season with Worcestershire sauce, garlic powder, salt, and pepper.

Preheat the Air Fryer at 400°F for 4 minutes.

Spread the steak and potatoes in an even layer in an air fryer basket. Air fry at 400°F for 10-18 minutes, shaking and flipping and the steak and potatoes about 3 times through the cooking process (time depends on your preferred doneness, the thickness of the steak, and size of air fryer).

Check the steak to see how well done it is cooked. If you want the steak more done, add an extra 2-5 minutes of cooking time.

Garnish with parsley and drizzle with optional melted butter and/or optional chili flakes. Season with additional salt & pepper if desired. Serve warm

Nutrition

Calories: 321kcal | Carbohydrates: 8g | Protein: 24g | Fat: 22g | Saturated Fat: 11g | Cholesterol: 84mg | Sodium: 130mg | Potassium: 550mg | Fiber: 1g | Sugar: 1g | Vitamin A: 192IU | Vitamin C: 6mg | Calcium: 25mg | Iron: 4mg

Perfect Air Fryer Steak

Prep Time: 20 minutes

Cook Time: 12 minutes

Resting Time: 5 minutes

Total Time: 32 minutes

Servings: 2

Ingredients

- 2 8 oz Ribeye steak
- Salt
- Freshly cracked black pepper
- Olive oil
- Garlic Butter
- 1 stick unsalted butter softened
- 2 tbsp fresh parsley chopped
- 2 tsp garlic minced
- 1 tsp Worcestershire Sauce
- 1/2 tsp salt

Instructions

Prepare Garlic Butter by mixing butter, parsley garlic, Worcestershire sauce, and salt until thoroughly combined.

Place in parchment paper and roll into a log. Refrigerate until ready to use.

Remove steak from the fridge and allow to sit at room temperature for 20 minutes. Rub a little bit of olive oil on both sides of the steak and season with salt and freshly cracked black pepper.

Grease your Air Fryer basket by rubbing a little bit of oil on the basket. Preheat Air Fryer to 400 degrees Fahrenheit. Once preheated, place steaks in the air fryer and cook for 12 minutes, flipping halfway through.

Remove from air fryer and allow to rest for 5 minutes. Top with garlic butter.

Nutrition

Calories: 683kcal

Air Fryer Steak

Prep Time: 5 min

Cook Time: 12 min

Total Time: 12 min

Yield: 2

Ingredients

- 2 (1 in thick) Steaks Rib Eye, or Tri-Tip), 4 to 6 oz each
- Salt and Pepper to taste
- 2 tablespoons of butter (optional)

Instructions

If your air fryer re□uires preheating, preheat your air fryer. Set the temperature to 400 degrees Fahrenheit.

Season your steak with salt and pepper on each side.

Place the steak in your air fryer basket. Do not overlap the steaks.

Medium Steak: Set the time to 12 minutes and flip the steak at 6.

Medium Rare: For a medium-rare steak, cook the steak for 10 minutes and flip it at 5 minutes.

Nutrition

Serving Size: 4|Calories: 250|Sodium: 60|Fat: 17|Saturated Fat: 7|Carbohydrates: 0|Fiber: 0|Protein: 23

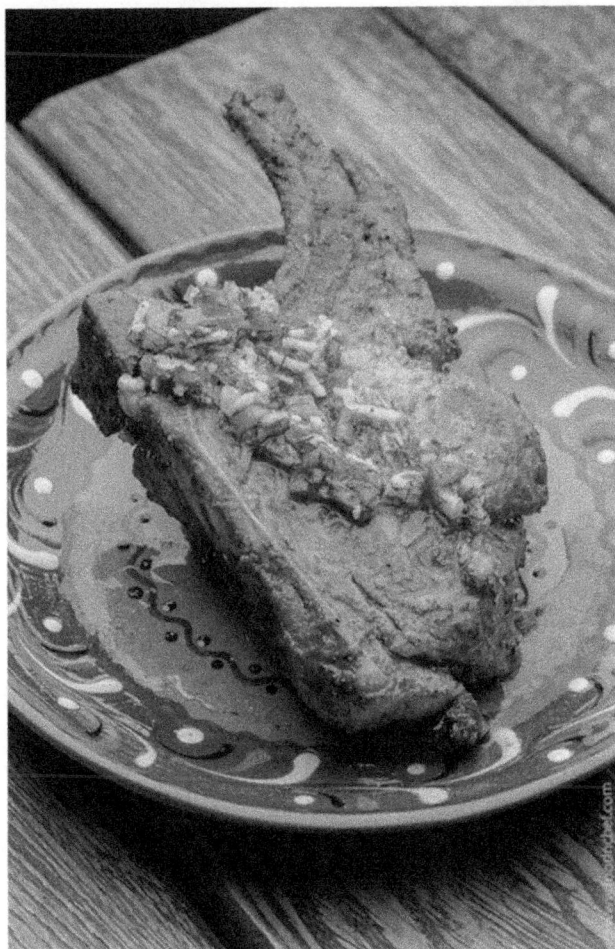

Air Fryer Steak

Prep Time: 5 Minutes

Cook Time: 8 Minutes

Rest Time: 5 Minutes

Total Time: 18 Minutes

Servings: 2 Steaks

Ingredients

- 2 steaks 1" thick, ribeye, sirloin, or striploin
- 1 tablespoon olive oil
- 1 tablespoon salted butter melted
- Steak seasoning to taste

Instructions

Remove steaks from the fridge at least 30 minutes before cooking. Preheat air fryer to 400°F.

Rub the steaks with olive oil and melted butter. Generously season on each side.

Add the steaks to the air fryer basket and cook for 8-12 minutes (flipping after 4 minutes) or until steaks reach desired doneness.

Remove steaks from the air fryer and transfer them to a plate. Rest at least 5 minutes before serving. Top with additional butter if desired and serve.

Nutrition Information

Calories: 582, Carbohydrates: 1g, Protein: 46g, Fat: 45g, Saturated Fat: 19g, Cholesterol: 153mg, Sodium: 168mg, Potassium: 606mg, Sugar: 1g, Vitamin A: 209IU, Calcium: 16mg, Iron: 4mg

Air Fryer Roast Beef With Herb Crust

Prep Time: 5 minutes

Cook Time: 1 hour

RestingTime: 10 minutes

Total Time: 1 hour 15 minutes

Servings: 6 people

Ingredients

- 2- 2-pound beef roast
- 2 teaspoons garlic powder
- 2 teaspoons onion salt
- 2 teaspoons parsley
- 2 teaspoons thyme
- 2 teaspoons basil 1/2 tablespoon salt 1 teaspoon pepper
- 1 tablespoon olive oil

Instructions

Preheat the air fryer for 15 minutes at 390 degrees.

Combine the garlic powder, onion salt, parsley, thyme, and basil, salt, and pepper. Rub the roast with olive oil then rub the herb mixture over the entire roast.

Place the roast in the preheated air fryer. Set timer for 15 minutes. After 15 minutes, remove the basket and turn the roast over.

Reduce the temperature to 360 degrees on the air fryer and return the roast. Cook for another 60 minutes, or until the thermometer reaches desired degree of doneness.

Let roast rest for 15 minutes before slicing.

Nutrition

Calories: 336kcal | Carbohydrates: 1g | Protein: 69g | Fat: 16g | Saturated Fat: 5.5g | Cholesterol: 136mg

Air Fryer Garlic Steak Bites

Prep Time: 10 Minutes

Cook Time: 15 Minutes

Total Time: 25 Minutes

Servings: 4 People

Ingredients

- 1 pound New York steak or sirloin steak cut into one inch cubes
- 2 Tablespoons olive oil
- 1/2 teaspoon salt
- 1/4 teaspoon pepper
- 1 teaspoon Italian seasoning
- 3 cloves garlic minced

Herb Butter:

- 1/4 cup butter melted
- 1/2 teaspoon thyme
- 1/2 teaspoon rosemary minced
- 1 teaspoon parsley minced

Instructions

In a medium-sized bowl add the steak bites, olive oil, salt, pepper, Italian seasoning, and garlic. Add to the basket of the air fryer.

Cook at 400 degrees for 10-12 minutes. Once cooked toss to coat with the garlic herb butter.

Nutrition Facts

Calories: 169kcal Carbohydrates: 1g Protein: 1g

Fat: 19g Saturated Fat: 8g Cholesterol: 31mg Sodium: 393mg Potassium: 9mg Fiber: 1g Sugar: 1g Calcium: 15mg Iron: 1mg

Best Air Fryer Steak Recipe

Prep Time: 15 minutes

Cook Time: 10 minutes

Total Time: 25 minutes

Servings: 2

Ingredients

- 2 Steak Ribeye, New York, Sirloin, or any steak of choice.
- 1 teaspoon Paprika
- 1/2 teaspoon Oregano
- 1/2 teaspoon Black pepper or to taste
- Salt

For the Garlic Herb Butter

- 2 tablespoons Butter
- 1 teaspoon garlic granules
- 1 tablespoon freshly chopped Parsley

Instructions

Add the paprika, oregano, black pepper, salt to a bowl and mix.

Add the garlic granules and freshly chopped parsley in the butter, mix well and store in the fridge till it's time to use.

Garlic herb butter displayed.

Pat steak dry and season both sides with the seasoning mix. Leave to marinate for 10-15 minutes. Seasoned steaks.

Arrange the side of the steak by side in the air fryer basket and air fry at a temperature of 195C for 10 minutes (well done). After half of the time, bring the air fryer basket out and turn the steak to the other side.

Steaks displayed in the air fryer basket.

After the 5 minutes cycle is done, bring the steaks out, serve and immediately add the garlic butter to the steaks.

Enjoy air fryer garlic butter steak.

Air fryer steak topped with garlic butter.

Nutrition Information

Calories: 581kcal | Carbohydrates: 2g | Protein: 46g | Fat: 43g | Saturated Fat: 21g | Cholesterol: 168mg

| Sodium: 219mg | Potassium: 646mg | Fiber: 1g | Sugar: 1g | Vitamin A: 876IU | Calcium: 24mg | Iron: 4mg

Perfect Air Fryer Steak: Paleo, Whole30, Keto, Easy!

Prep Time: 5 Mins

Cook Time: 12 Mins

Total Time: 17 Mins

Ingredients

- 2 sirloin steaks
- 2–3 tbsp steak seasoning
- Spray oil or cooking fat of choice (I prefer avocado oil)

Instructions

First, pat the steak dry and let come to room temperature Spray (or brush) oil lightly on the steak and season liberally

Spray or coat the bottom of the air fryer basket with oil and place the steaks into the air fryer. The steaks can be touching or sort of "smooshed" in the basket.

Cook at 400 degrees F. for 6 minutes, flip the steaks, and cook for another 6 minutes. If you want your steak more well-done, add 2-3 minutes. Let rest before serving.

Nutritional Value

Calories: 195kcal | Carbohydrates: 5g | Protein: 12g |Saturated Fat: 6g | Cholesterol:44mg | Sodium: 43mg | Potassium: 321mg | Fiber: 2g | Sugar: 1g | Calcium: 15mg | Iron: 3mg

How To Make Steak In The Air Fryer

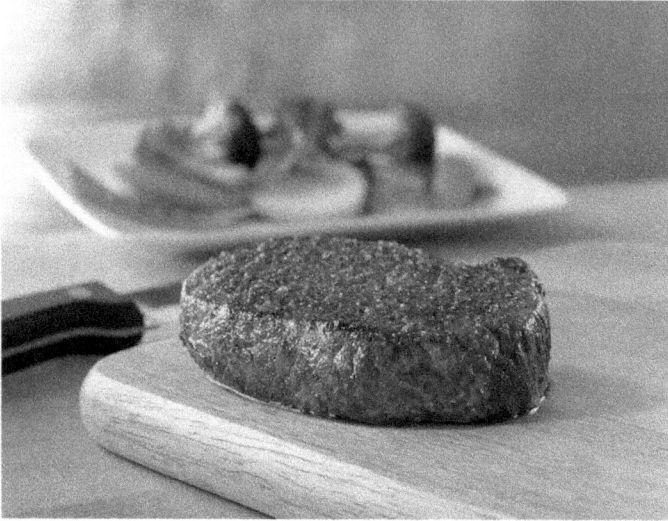

Prep Time: 5 Minutes

Cook Time: 15 Minutes

Total Time: 20 Minutes

Ingredients

- 2 Pounds Steak (I Used Delmonico)
- Salt
- Pepper
- Garlic Powder
- 2 Tbs Butter

Instructions

Preheat your air fryer to 400 for about 5 minutes Salt and pepper both sides of the steak

Place a pad of butter on top of each steak Place on the top rack of your air fryer

Cook on-air fry for 15 minutes for medium-well Flip over after 7 minutes

For Medium-rare cook for 10 minutes flipping after 5

For well-done cook for 20 minutes flipping after 10 minutes Remove steak and let rest for 5 minutes and serve

Nutrition Information:

Calories: 1371| Total Fat: 95g| Saturated Fat: 40g| Trans Fat: 0g| Unsaturated Fat: 41g| Cholesterol: 471mg| Sodium: 619mg| Carbohydrates: 2g| Fiber: 0g| Sugar: 0g| Protein: 119g

Air Fryer Steak Bites With Mushrooms

Prep Time: 10 mins

Cook Time: 15 mins

Total Time: 25 mins

Ingredients

- 2 lb beef
- 2 lb mushrooms
- 2 tbsp Worcester sauce
- 1 tbsp salt
- 1 tbsp pepper

Instructions

Preheat an Air Fryer for 3 minutes at 400 °F. Cut beef into bite-size pieces and mushrooms into halves. Mushrooms and steak in a bowl

Add Worchester sauce, salt, and pepper to the mixture. Let it sit for a few minutes. Steak and mushrooms withs seasoning

Add beef and mushrooms to the air fryer basket. Air-dry it for 5 minutes. Uncooked steak and mushrooms in a basket

Remove the basket and toss the steak bites to ensure all the sides are getting nice and crispy. Basket with steak and mushrooms

Air fry for another 5-7 minutes. Once complete, check to make sure the temperature of the beef reached 145F.

Steak bites with mushrooms in an air fryer basket

Nutrition Facts

Fat: 31g Saturated Fat: 12g Cholesterol: 107mg Sodium: 1327mg Potassium: 948mg Carbohydrates: 7g Fiber: 2g

Sugar: 4g Protein: 31g Vitamin C: 4mg Calcium: 42mg Iron: 4mg

Air Fryer Steak

Ready In: 49min

Prep Time: 15min

Cook Time: 9min

Ingredients

- 2 boneless ribeye steaks
- 1 tablespoon steak rub
- 1 teaspoon kosher salt
- 1 tablespoon unsalted butter

Directions

Rub steaks with steak rub and salt. Allow resting at room temperature for 15 to 30 minutes. The longer you allow them to rest with the rub on, the more flavorful they will be!

Preheat air fryer for 5 minutes at 400°F (200°C).

Arrange steaks in a single layer in an air fryer basket, work in batches as needed and cook about 9 minutes for medium-rare. The internal temperature should read at least 145°F (63°C).

Transfer steak to a cutting board and put half the butter on each steak. Allow resting for at least 5 minutes before slicing into 1/2-inch thick slices.

Nutrition Facts

Calories: 301; 23g Fat; 0.0g Carbohydrates; 23g Protein; 88mg Cholesterol; 1111mg Sodium.

Air Fryer Italian-Style Meatballs

Active Time: 10 Mins

Total Time: 45 Mins

Yield: Serves 12 (2 meatballs)

Ingredients

- 2 tablespoons olive oil
- 1 medium shallot, minced (about 2 Tbsp.)
- 3 cloves garlic, minced (about 1 Tbsp.)
- 1/4 cup whole-wheat panko crumbs
- 2 tablespoons whole milk
- 2/3 pound lean ground beef
- 1/3 pound bulk turkey sausage
- 1 large egg, lightly beaten
- 1/4 cup finely chopped fresh flat-leaf parsley
- 1 tablespoon chopped fresh rosemary
- 1 tablespoon finely chopped fresh thyme
- 1 tablespoon Dijon mustard
- 1/2 teaspoon kosher salt

How To Make It

Preheat air-fryer to 400°F. Heat oil in a medium nonstick pan over medium-high heat. Add shallot and cook until softened, 1 to 2 minutes. Add garlic and cook just until fragrant, 1 minute. Remove from heat.

In a large bowl, combine panko and milk. Let stand 5 minutes.

Add cooked shallot and garlic to the panko mixture, along with beef, turkey sausage egg, parsley, rosemary, thyme, mustard, and salt. Stir to gently combine.

Gently shape mixture into 1 1/2-inch ball. Place shaped balls in a single-layer in the air-fryer basket. Cook half the meatballs at 400°F until lightly browned and cooked for 10 to 11 minutes. Remove and keep warm. Repeat with remaining meatballs.

Serve warm meatballs with toothpicks as an appetizer or serve over pasta, rice, or spiralized zoodles for a main dish.

Nutritional Information

Calories: 122| Fat: 8g| Sat fat: 2g| Unsatfat: 5g| Protein: 10g| Carbohydrate| 0g Fiber 0g| Sugars 0g| Added sugars: 0g| Sodium: 254mg

Air Fryer Marinated Steak

Prep Time: 5 minutes

Cook Time: 10 minutes

Total Time: 15 minutes

Servings: 2

Ingredients

- 2 New York Strip Steaks (mine were about 6-8 oz each) You can use any cut of steak
- 1 tablespoon low-sodium soy sauce This is used to provide liquid to marinate the meat and make it juicy.
- 1 teaspoon liquid smoke or a cap full
- 1 tablespoon mccormick's Grill Mates Montreal Steak Seasoning or Steak Rub (or season to taste) See recipe notes for instructions on how to create your steak rub
- 1/2 tablespoon unsweetened cocoa powder
- Salt and pepper to taste
- Melted butter (optional)

Instructions

Drizzle the steak with soy sauce and liquid smoke. You can do this inside Ziploc bags if you wish. Season the steak with the seasonings.

Refrigerate for at least a couple of hours, preferably overnight.

Place the steak in the air fryer. I did not use any oil. Cook two steaks at a time (if the air fryer is the standard size). You can use an accessory grill pan, a layer rack, or the standard air fryer basket.

Cook for 5 minutes at 370 degrees. After 5 minutes, open the air fryer and examine your steak. Cook time will vary depending on your desired doneness. Use a meat thermometer and cook to 125° F for rare, 135° F for medium-rare, 145° F for medium, 155° F for medium-well, and 160° F for well done.

I cooked the steak for an additional 2 minutes for medium-done steak. Remove the steak from the air fryer and drizzle with melted butter.

Nutrition

Serving: 0.5steak | Calories: 476kcal | Carbohydrates: 1g | Protein: 49g | Fat: 28g

Air Fryer Steak Bites And Mushrooms

Prep Time: 1 hour 5 minutes

Cook Time: 15 minutes

Total Time: 1 hour 20 minutes

Servings: 2

Ingredients

- 1 teaspoon kosher salt
- 1/2 teaspoon garlic powder
- 1/4 teaspoon black pepper
- 2 Tablespoons Worcestershire Sauce
- 2 Tablespoons avocado oil (Click here for my favorite brand on Amazon)
- 8 oz Baby Bella Mushrooms, sliced
- 1 pound Top Sirloin steak, cut into 1.5 inch cubes

Instructions

Combine all your ingredients for the marinade into a large mixing bowl.

Add your steak cubes and sliced mushrooms into your mixing bowl with the marinade and toss to coat. Let the steak and mushrooms marinate for 1 hour.

Preheat your Air Fryer to 400F for 5 minutes.

Make sure you spray the inside of your air fryer will a cooking spray and pour your steak and mushrooms into the air fryer basket.

Cook the steak and mushrooms in the Air Fryer for 5 minutes at 400F. Open the basket and shake the steak and mushrooms so they cook evenly. Continue to cook for 5 minutes more.

Check the steak using an internal meat thermometer. If the steak has not reached your desired doneness, continue to cook in 3-minute intervals until the thermometer placed in the center of 1 steak bite reaches the desired temperature. (Rare=125F, Medium-rare=130F, Medium=140F, Medium- well=150F, well-done=160F)

Serve

Nutritional Value

Calories: 572kcal | Carbohydrates: 1g | Protein: 46g | Fat: 43g | Saturated Fat: 22g | Cholesterol: 168mg | Sodium: 219mg | Potassium: 606mg | Sugar: 1g | Calcium: 16mg | Iron: 4mg

Air Fryer Beef Tips

Prep Time 2 minutes

Cook Time 12 minutes

Marinate Time 5 minutes

Total Time 14 minutes

Servings: 4

Ingredients

- 1 pound ribeye or New York steak, cut into 1-inch cubes
- 2 tsp sea salt
- 1 tsp black pepper
- 1 tsp garlic powder
- 2 tsp onion powder
- 1 tsp paprika
- 2 tsp rosemary crushed
- 2 tbsp coconut aminos

Instructions

Place steak cubes in a medium sized bowl.

In a small bowl, combine the salt, pepper, garlic powder, onion powder, paprika, and rosemary. Mix well.

Sprinkle the mixed dry seasoning on the steak cubes. Mix to evenly distribute the seasoning. Sprinkle the coconut aminos all over the seasoned steak. Mix well.

Let it sit for 5 minutes.

Place the steak in a single layer in the air fryer basket. Cook at 380F for 12 minutes.

Shake the basket halfway to ensure that the steak cooks evenly.

Remove from the air fryer and let it cool for a few minutes before serving.

Nutritional Value

Total fat: 3.7g sodium: 1820.8mg sugar: 11.3g Vitamin A: 169.2ug

Carbohydrates: 33.6mg Protein:18g

Vitamin C: 165.5mg

Air Fryer Beef Kabobs

Prep Time: 30 minutes

Cook Time: 8 minutes

Servings: 4 servings

Ingredients

- 1.5 pounds sirloin steak cut into 1-inch chunks
- 1 large bell pepper color of choice
- 1 large red onion or onion of choice

For The Marinade:

- 4 tablespoons olive oil
- 2 cloves garlic minced
- 1 tablespoon lemon juice
- 1/2 teaspoon
- 1/2 teaspoon
- Salt and pepper pinch

Instructions

In a large bowl, combine the beef and ingredients for the marinade until fully combined. Cover and marinate in the fridge for 30 minutes or up to 24 hours.

When ready to cook, preheat the air fryer to 400F. Thread the beef, pepper, and onion onto skewers. Place skewers into the preheated air fryer and the air fryer for 8-10 minutes, turning halfway through until charred on the outside and tender on the inside.

Nutrition

Calories: 382kcal | Carbohydrates: 6g | Protein: 38g | Fat: 22g | Saturated Fat: 5g | Cholesterol: 104mg | Sodium: 105mg | Potassium: 708mg | Fiber: 1g | Sugar: 3g | Vitamin A: 1358IU | Vitamin C: 56mg | Calcium: 60mg | Iron: 3mg

Air Fryer Corned Beef

Total Time: 2 hours

Ingredients

- Corned Beef, 3-4 pounds
- 1/2 Cup Brown Sugar
- 1/4 cup Dijon Mustard
- 1 TBSP Apple Cider Vinegar

Instructions

Mix brown sugar, Dijon mustard, & apple cider vinegar together. Baste corned beef with glaze and tightly wrap it in aluminum foil. Air Fry at 360 degrees for 1 hour.

Unwrap aluminum foil, baste again, and loosely wrap with aluminum foil. Air Fry at 360 degrees for 40 minutes.

Remove foil, baste one last time. Air Fry at 400 degrees for 10 minutes.

Nutrition Information:

Total Fat: 8g|Saturated Fat: 3g|Trans Fat: 0g|Unsaturated Fat: 5g|Cholesterol: 42mg|Sodium: 688mg|Carbohydrates: 16g|Fiber: 0g|Sugar: 15g|Protein: 8g

Air Fryer Ground Beef

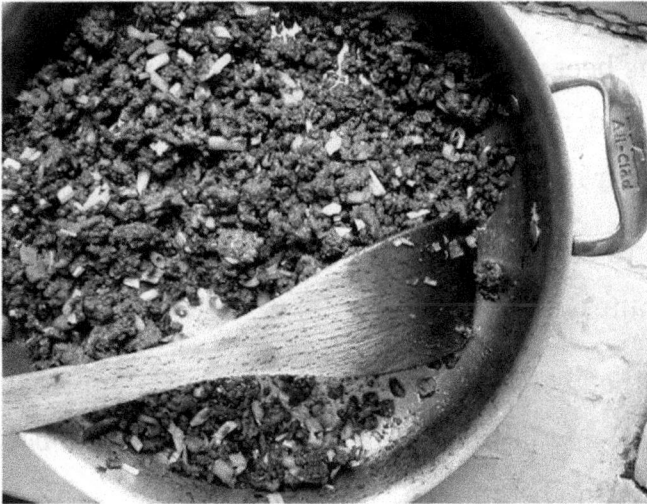

Prep Time: 2 minutes

Cook Time: 10 minutes

Yield: 6 servings

Ingredients

- 1 to 1 and 1/2 lbs. ground beef
- 1 tsp. salt
- 1/2 tsp. pepper
- 1/2 tsp. garlic powder

Instructions

Put the ground beef into the basket of the air fryer.

Season the beef with salt, pepper, and garlic powder. Stir it a bit with a wooden spoon. Cook in the air fryer at 400°F for 5 minutes. Stir it around.

Continue to cook until cooked through and no longer pink, 3-5 more minutes.

Crumble the beef up using a wooden spoon. Remove the basket and discard any fat and liquid left behind. Use the beef in your favorite ground beef recipe.

Nutritional Value

Total Fat: 7.5g Sodium: 437.5mg Sugar: 0g Vitamin A: 3.1ug

Carbohydrates: 0.3g Protein: 15.1g

Air Fryer Steak With Easy Herb Butter

Prep Time: 6 Mins

Cook Time: 9 Mins

Total Time: 15 Mins

Ingredients

- 2 medium steaks about 8 ounces each
- 2 teaspoon salt
- Herb butter
- 1/4 cup butter softened
- 1 clove garlic
- 1/4 teaspoon salt minced
- 1 tablespoon parsley chopped
- Pepper lots, to taste
- Wine pairings
- 2018 adelante pinot noir 2017 hushkeeper zinfandel
- 2018 middle jane cabernet sauvignon reserve

Instructions

Mix butter, garlic, salt, parsley, and pepper together for herb butter. Shape into a log. Chill in the fridge. (See notes.)

Preheat the air fryer for 5 minutes at 400° F. Liberally salt both sides of the steak. Add the steaks and cook for 7-9 minutes for medium-rare.

Immediately remove from air fryer. Rest 5 minutes.

Nutrition

Calories: 678kcal Carbohydrates: 1g Protein: 46g

Fat: 55g

Saturated Fat: 29g Cholesterol: 199mg Sodium: 2938mg Potassium: 608mg Sugar: 1g

Vitamin A: 912IU Vitamin C: 3mg Calcium: 23mg Iron: 4mg

Net Carbs: 1g

Air Fryer Roast Beef

Prep Time: 5 Minutes

Cook Time: 45 Minutes

Inactive Time: 10 Minutes

Total Time: 1 Hour

Ingredients

- 2 lb beef roast
- 1 tbsp olive oil
- 1medium onion, (optional)
- 1 tsp salt
- 2 tsp rosemary and thyme, (fresh or dried)

Instructions

Preheat air fryer to 390°F (200°C).

Mix sea salt, rosemary, and oil on a plate.

Pat the beef roast dry with paper towels. Place beef roast on a plate and turn so that the oil-herb mix coats the outside of the beef.

Seasoned beef roast on a white plate

If using, peel the onion and cut it in half, place onion halves in the air fryer basket. Place beef roast in the air fryer basket.

Beef roast in the air fryer basket Set to air fry beef for 15 minutes.

When the time is up, change the temperature to 360°F (180°C). Some air fryers re?uire you to turn food during cooking, so check your manual and turn the beef roast over if required (my Philips Viva air fryer doesn't need food to be turned).

Set the beef to cook for an additional 30 minutes. This should give you medium-rare beef. Though is best to monitor the temperature with a meat thermometer to ensure that it is cooked to your liking. Cook for additional 5-minute intervals if you prefer it more well done.

Remove roast beef from the air fryer, cover with kitchen foil and leave to rest for at least ten minutes before serving. This allows the meat to finish cooking and the juices to reabsorb into the meat.

Carve the roast beef thinly against the grain and serve with roasted or steamed vegetables, wholegrain mustard, and gravy.

Nutrition Information:

Calories: 212| Total Fat: 7g| Saturated Fat: 2g| Unsaturated Fat: 0g| Cholesterol: 83mg| Sodium: 282mg| Carbohydrates: 2g| Fiber: 1g| Sugar: 1g| Protein: 33g

Air Fryer Chicken Fried Steak

Prep Time: 20 minutes

Cook Time: 8 minutes

Total Time: 28 minutes

Ingredients

For The Steaks

- 2 cube steaks, 5-6 ounces each
- 3/4 cup All-Purpose Flour
- 1 teaspoon Ground Black Pepper
- 1 teaspoon Kosher Salt
- 1/2 teaspoon smoked paprika
- 1/2 teaspoon Onion Powder
- 1/2 teaspoon garlic powder
- 1/4 teaspoon Cayenne Pepper
- 2 teaspoons crumbled dried sage
- 3/4 cup buttermilk
- 1 teaspoon hot pepper sauce
- 1 Egg
- Non-Stick Cooking Spray

For The Gravy

- 4 tablespoons butter
- 2 tablespoons All-Purpose Flour
- 1 teaspoon Cracked Black Pepper
- 1/2 teaspoon Kosher Salt
- 1/4 teaspoon garlic salt
- 1/2 cup Whole Milk
- 1/2 cup Heavy Cream

Instructions

Steaks

For the flour dredge, mix together in a shallow bowl, whisk the flour, 1 teaspoon pepper, 1 teaspoon salt, paprika, onion powder, garlic powder, cayenne, and sage.

In a separate shallow bowl, whisk the buttermilk, hot pepper sauce, and egg.

Pat the steaks dry with a paper towel. Season to taste with salt and pepper. Allow standing for 5 minutes, then pat dry again with a paper towel.

Dredge the steaks in the seasoned flour mixture, shaking off any excess. Then dredge in the buttermilk mixture, allowing excess to drip off. Dredge in the flour mixture again, shaking off excess. Place the breaded steaks on a sheet pan and press any remaining flour mixture onto the steaks, making sure that each steak is completely coated. Let stand for 10 minutes.

Place steaks in the air fryer basket. Lightly coat with vegetable oil spray. Set the air fryer to 400°F for 8 minutes, carefully turning steaks and coating the other side with vegetable oil spray halfway through the cooking time.

Gravy

Meanwhile, for the gravy: In a small saucepan, melt the butter over low heat. Whisk in the flour, pepper, salt, and garlic salt, continually whisking.

Slowly add the milk and cream mixture, whisking constantly. Turn the heat to medium and cook, whisking occasionally, until thickened.

Use a meat thermometer to ensure the steaks have reached an internal temperature of 145°F. Serve the steaks topped with the gravy.

Nutrition Facts

Calories: 787kcal | Carbohydrates: 54g | Protein: 51g | Fat: 40g | Fiber: 2g | Sugar: 11g

Air Fryer Korean BBQ Beef

Prep Time: 15 Minutes

Cook Time: 30 Minutes

Total Time: 45 Minutes

Ingredients

Meat

- 1 Pound Flank Steak or Thinly Sliced Steak
- 1/4 Cup Corn Starch
- Pompeian Oils Coconut Spray

Sauce

- 1/2 Cup Soy Sauce or Gluten-Free Soy Sauce
- 1/2 Cup Brown Sugar
- 2 Tbsp Pompeian White Wine Vinegar
- 1 Clove Garlic, Crushed
- 1 Tbsp Hot Chili Sauce
- 1 Tsp Ground Ginger
- 1/2 Tsp Sesame Seeds 1 Tbsp Cornstarch
- 1 Tbsp Water

Instructions

Begin by preparing the steak. Thinly slice it then toss in the cornstarch. Spray the basket or line it with foil in the air fryer with coconut oil spray. Add the steak and spray another coat of spray on top.

Cook in the air fryer for 10 minutes at 390*, turn the steak, and cook for an additional 10 minutes. While the steak is cooking add the sauce ingredients EXCEPT for the cornstarch and water to a medium saucepan.

Warm it up to a low boil, then whisk in the cornstarch and water. Carefully remove the steak and pour the sauce over the steak, mix well. Serve topped with sliced green onions, cooked rice, and green beans.

Nutrition Information

Total Fat: 22g| Saturated Fat: 10g| Trans Fat: 0g| Unsaturated Fat: 10g|Cholesterol: 113mg| Sodium: 1531mg| Carbohydrates: 32g| Fiber: 2g| Sugar: 21g| Protein: 39g

Air Fryer Mongolian Beef

Prep Time: 20 Minutes

Cook Time: 20 Minutes

Total Time: 40 Minutes

Ingredients

Meat

- 1 Lb Flank Steak
- 1/4 Cup Corn Starch

Sauce

- 2 Tsp Vegetable Oil
- 1/2 Tsp Ginger
- 1 Tbsp Minced Garlic
- 1/2 Cup Soy Sauce or Gluten Free Soy Sauce
- 1/2 Cup Water
- 3/4 Cup Brown Sugar Packed

Extras

- Cooked Rice Green Beans Green Onions

Instructions

Thinly slice the steak into long pieces, then coat with the corn starch.

Place in the Air Fryer and cook on 390* for 5 minutes on each side. (Start with 5 minutes and add more time if needed. I cook this for 10 minutes on each side; however, others have suggested that was too long for theirs.)

While the steak cooks, warm up all sauce ingredients in a medium sized saucepan on medium-high heat.

Whisk the ingredients together until it gets to a low boil.

Once both the steak and sauce are cooked, place the steak in a bowl with the sauce and let it soak in for about 5-10 minutes.

When ready to serve, use tongs to remove the steak and let the excess sauce drip off. Place steak on cooked rice and green beans, top with additional sauce if you prefer.

Nutrition Information:

Total Fat: 16g| Saturated Fat: 5g| Trans Fat: 0g| Unsaturated Fat: 8g| Cholesterol: 116mg| Sodium: 2211mg| Carbohydrates: 57g| Fiber: 1g| Sugar: 35g| Protein: 44g

Air Fryer Beef And Bean Taquitos

Prep Time: 10 Minutes

Cook Time: 15 Minutes

Total Time: 25 Minutes

Ingredients

- 1 Pound Ground Beef
- 1 Package Gluten-Free or Regular Taco Seasoning
- 1 Can of Refried Beans
- 1 Cup Shredded Sharp Cheddar
- 20 White Corn Tortillas

Instructions

Begin by preparing the ground beef if it isn't already.

Brown the meat on medium-high heat and add in the taco seasoning per the instructions on the package.

Once you are done with the meat, heat up the corn tortillas for about 30 seconds.

Spray the air fryer basket with non-stick cooking spray or add a sheet of foil and spray. Add ground beef, beans, and a bit of cheese to each tortilla.

Wrap them tightly and place seam side down in the air fryer.

Add a quick spray of cooking oil spray, such as olive oil cooking spray. Cook at 390 degrees for 12 minutes.

Repeat for any additional tortillas.

Nutrition Information:

Total Fat: 9g| Saturated Fat: 4g| Trans Fat: 0g| Unsaturated Fat: 4g| Cholesterol: 31mg| Sodium: 207mg| Carbohydrates: 14g| Fiber: 2g| Sugar: 0g| Protein: 11g

Air Fryer Steak Fajitas With Onions And Peppers

Prep Time: 10 Minutes

Cook Time: 15 Minutes

Total Time: 25 Minutes

Ingredients

- 1 lb Thin Cut Steak
- 1 Green Bell Pepper Sliced
- 1 Yellow Bell Pepper Sliced
- 1 Red Bell Pepper Sliced
- 1/2 Cup White Onions Sliced
- 1 Packet Gluten Free Fajita Seasoning
- Olive Oil Spray
- Gluten-Free Corn Tortillas or Flour Tortillas

Instructions

Line the basket of the air fryer with foil and coat with spray.

Thinly slice the steak against the grain, this should be about 1/4 inch slices. Mix the steak with peppers and onions.

Add to the air fryer.

Evenly coat with the fajita seasoning. Cook for 5 minutes on 390*.

Mix up the steak mixture.

Continue cooking for an additional 5-10 minutes until your desired doneness. Serve in warm tortillas.

Nutrition Information:

Total Fat: 17g| Saturated Fat: 6g| Trans Fat: 0g| Unsaturated Fat: 9g| Cholesterol: 73mg| Sodium: 418mg| Carbohydrates: 15g| Fiber: 2g| Sugar: 4g| Protein: 22g

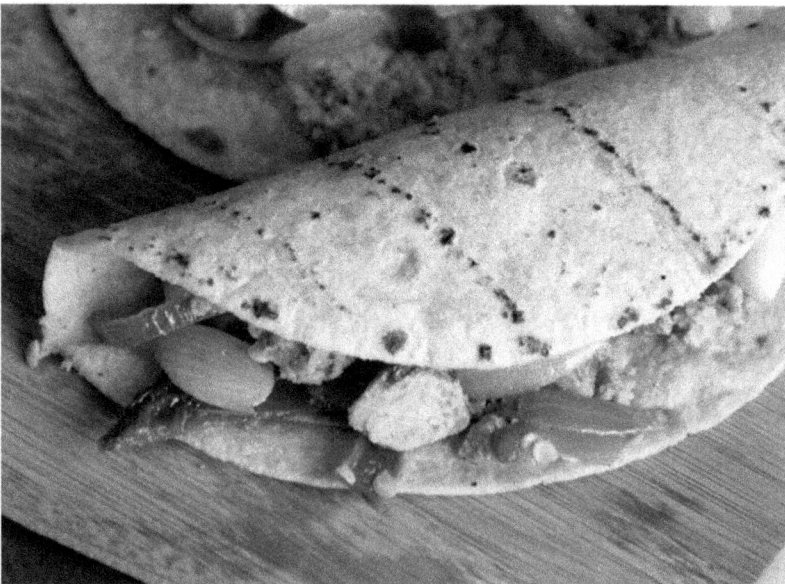

Air Fryer Meatballs (Low Carb)

Prep Time: 10 minutes

Cook Time: 14 minutes

Total Time: 24 minutes

Servings: 3 -4

Ingredients

- 1 lb Lean Ground Beef
- 1/4 Cup Marinara Sauce
- 1 Tablespoon Dried Minced Onion or Freeze Dried Shallots
- 1 teaspoon Minced Garlic I used freeze-dried
- 1 teaspoon Pizza Seasoning or Italian Seasoning
- 1/3 Cup Shredded Parmesan
- 1 Egg
- Salt and Pepper to taste
- Shredded Mozzarella Cheese optional
- 1 1/4 cups Marinara Sauce optional

Instructions

Mix together all ingredients except reserve 1 1/4 cup of the marinara sauce and the mozzarella cheese. Form mixture into 12 meatballs and place in a single layer in the air fryer basket.

Cook in the air fryer at 350 for 11 minutes.

Optional: Place meatballs in an air fryer pan, toss in remaining marinara sauce, and top with mozzarella cheese. Place air fryer pan into the basket and cook at 350 for 3 minutes.

Nutritional Value

Calories: 572kcal | Carbohydrates: 1g | Protein: 46g | Fat: 43g | Saturated Fat: 22g | Cholesterol: 168mg

| Sodium: 219mg | Potassium: 606mg | Sugar: 1g | Vitamin A: 355IU | Calcium: 16mg | Iron: 4mg

Air Fryer Roast Beef

Prep Time: 5 mins

Cook Time: 35 mins

Total Time: 40 mins

Ingredients

- 2 lb beef roast top round or eye of round is best
- Oil for spraying
- Rub
- 1 tbs kosher salt
- 1 tsp black pepper
- 2 tsp garlic powder
- 1 tsp summer savory or thyme

Instructions

Mix all rub ingredients and rub into the roast.

Place fat side down in the basket of the air fryer (or set up for rotisserie if your air fryer is so e?uipped) Lightly spray with oil.

Set fryer to 400 degrees F and air fry for 20 minutes; turn fat-side up and spray lightly with oil. Continue cooking for 15 additional minutes at 400 degrees F.

Remove the roast from the fryer, tent with foil, and let the meat rest for 10 minutes.

The time given should produce a rare roast which should be 125 degrees F on a meat thermometer. Additional time will be needed for medium, medium-well, and well. Always use a meat thermometer to test the temperature.

Approximate times for medium and well respectively are 40 minutes and 45 minutes. Remember to always use a meat thermometer as times are approximate and fryers differ by wattage.

Nutrition

Calories: 238kcal | Carbohydrates: 1g | Protein: 25g | Fat: 14g | Saturated Fat: 6g | Cholesterol: 89mg | Sodium: 1102mg | Potassium: 448mg | Vitamin A: 55IU | Vitamin C: 0.3mg | Calcium: 37mg | Iron: 3mg

Air Fryer Stuffed Peppers

Prep Time: 15 Minutes

Cook Time: 15 Minutes

Total Time: 30 Minutes

Ingredients

- 6 Green Bell Peppers
- 1 Lb Lean Ground Beef
- 1 Tbsp Olive Oil
- 1/4 Cup Green Onion Diced
- 1/4 Cup Fresh Parsley
- 1/2 Tsp Ground Sage
- 1/2 Tsp Garlic Salt
- 1 Cup Cooked Rice
- 1 Cup Marinara Sauce More to Taste
- 1/4 Cup Shredded Mozzarella Cheese

Instructions

Warm-up a medium-sized skillet with the ground beef and cook until well done. Drain the beef and return to the pan.

Add in the olive oil, green onion, parsley, sage, and salt. Mix this well. Add in the cooked rice and marinara, mix well.

Cut the top off of each pepper and clean the seeds out.

Scoop the mixture into each of the peppers and place it in the basket of the air fryer. (I did 4 the first round, 2 the second to make them fit.)

Cook for 10 minutes at 355*, carefully open and add cheese.

Cook for an additional 5 minutes or until peppers are slightly soft and cheese is melted. Serve.

Nutrition Information

Total Fat: 13g| Saturated Fat: 4g| Trans Fat: 0g| Unsaturated Fat: 7g| Cholesterol: 70mg| Sodium: 419mg| Carbohydrates: 19g| Fiber: 2g| Sugar: 6g| Protein: 25g

Air Fryer Steak

Prep Time: 10 mins

Cook Time: 15 mins

Resting Time: 8 mins Total Time: 30 mins

Ingredients

- 2 (10 to 12 ounces EACH) sirloin steaks, about one inch thick, and at room temperature which is important for proper and even cooking.
- ½ tablespoon olive oil OR olive oil cooking spray, for the steaks
- 1 tablespoon kosher salt
- 1 tablespoon garlic powder
- 1 tablespoon onion powder
- ½ tablespoon paprika, sweet or smoked
- ½ tablespoon freshly ground black pepper
- 2 teaspoons dried herbs of choice

Instructions

Preheat Air Fryer to 400°F.

Rub both steaks with olive oil, or spray with cooking spray, and set aside.

In a small mixing bowl combine salt, garlic powder, onion powder, paprika, pepper, and dried herbs. This makes enough seasoning for about 4 large steaks.

Rub preferred amount of seasoning all over the steaks. Store leftover seasoning blends in a small airtight container and keeps it in a cool, dry place.

Place 1 steak in the Air Fryer basket and cook for 6 minutes at 400°F.

If you have a bigger Air Fryer, both steaks can fit in at the same time, but just make sure they aren't one on top of the other. You want a little space between the two.

Flip over the steak and continue to cook for 4 to 5 more minutes, or until cooked through.

Please use an Instant Read Thermometer to check for doneness; for a RARE steak, the temperature should register at 125°F to 130°F. For Medium-Rare, you want an internal temperature of 135°F.

IF the steak isn't cooked through, it may be too thick and you'll want to return the steak to the air fryer and give it a minute or two to finish cooking.

Repeat the cooking method with the other steak.

Remove from air fryer and let rest for 5 to 8 minutes before cutting. Serve with a pat of butter and garnish with chopped parsley.

Nutrition Facts

Fat: 17g Saturated Fat: 5g

Cholesterol: 173mg Sodium: 3656mg Potassium: 1112mg Carbohydrates: 8g Fiber: 2g

Sugar: 1g Protein: 64g Calcium: 99mg Iron: 5mg

Air Fryer Steak Fajitas

Prep Time: 10 mins

Cook Time: 10 mins

Total Time: 20 mins

Ingredients

- 2 pounds flank steak strips
- 1 packet taco seasoning
- 1/2 red bell pepper, seeded, cored, and sliced
- 1/2 yellow bell pepper, seeded, cored, and sliced
- 1 onion, peeled and sliced
- 2 tablespoons freshly squeezed lime juice
- Cooking spray
- Flour tortillas Cilantro, chopped

Instructions

Season steak with taco seasoning. Marinate for about 20 to 30 minutes.

Preheat your air fryer to 400 degrees. Spray the air fryer tray with cooking spray,

Arrange the seasoned beef on the air fryer tray, cooking in batches depending on the size of the air fryer.

Add a layer of the sliced onions and a layer of bell peppers on top of the meat.

Place in the air fryer for 10 minutes. Toss halfway through cooking to ensure the steak is cooked evenly.

Remove from the air fryer and drizzle with lime juice. Serve in warm tortillas with fresh cilantro.

Nutrition

Calories: 620kcal | Carbohydrates: 56g | Protein: 56g | Fat: 17g | Saturated Fat: 6g | Cholesterol: 136mg

| Sodium: 1446mg | Potassium: 1014mg | Fiber: 5g | Sugar: 8g | Vitamin A: 1350IU | Vitamin C: 55mg

| Calcium: 149mg | Iron: 7mg

Air Fryer Taco Calzones

Prep Time: 10 Minutes

Cook Time: 10 Minutes

Total Time: 20 Minutes

Ingredients

- 1 tube Pillsbury thin crust pizza dough
- 1 cup taco meat
- 1 cup shredded cheddar

Instructions

Spread out your sheet of pizza dough on a clean surface. Using a pizza cutter, cut the dough into 4 even squares.

Cut each square into a large circle using the pizza cutter. Set the dough scraps aside to make cinnamon sugar bites.

Top one half of each circle of dough with 1/4 cup taco meat and 1/4 cup shredded cheese.

Fold the empty half over the meat and cheese and press the edges of the dough together with a fork to seal it tightly. Repeat with all four calzones.

Gently pick up each calzone and spray it with pan spray or olive oil. Arrange them in your Air Fryer basket.

Cook the calzones at 325° for 8-10 minutes. Watch them closely at the 8-minute mark so you don't overcook them.

Serve with salsa and sour cream.

To make cinnamon sugar bites, cut the scraps of dough into even-sized pieces, about 2 inches long. Add them to the Air Fryer basket and cook at 325° for 5 minutes. Immediately toss with a 1:4 cinnamon-sugar mixture.

Nutrition Information

Total Fat: 31g| Saturated Fat: 14g| Trans Fat: 1g| Unsaturated Fat: 14g| Cholesterol: 58mg| Sodium: 814mg| Carbohydrates: 38g| Fiber: 2g| Sugar: 1g| Protein: 18g

Jalapeno Lime Air Fryer Steak

Prep Time: 5 mins

Cook Time: 10 mins

Marinate Time: 30 mins

Total Time: 45 mins

Servings: 4

Ingredients

- 1 lb flank steak used flat iron – check keywords
- 1 lime juice and zest
- 1 jalapeno, sliced
- 3 cloves of garlic, minced
- 1/2 cup fresh cilantro, roughly chopped
- 2 tablespoons light brown sugar
- 1/2 teaspoon paprika
- 1/2 teaspoon fresh cracked pepper
- 1/4 cup avocado oil
- Salt

Instructions

Preheat the air fryer to 400F.

Season the steak with salt and pepper. In a large mixing bowl, combine the avocado oil, paprika, pepper, brown sugar, cilantro, garlic, jalapeño, and lime zest from 1 lime. Add the steak and toss to coat. Marinate for 30 minutes.

Air fry for 10 minutes for medium-rare, flipping the steak halfway through. When the steak is finished cooking, squeeze lime juice from half a lime over it. Allow it to rest with the air fryer lid open for 10 minutes before slicing. Serve the steak with steamed veggies, over a salad, or in a taco.

Oven Instructions

To make the steak in the oven, preheat the broiler on high and cook for 6 minutes for medium-rare. Squeeze lime juice from half a lime over the steak and allow it to rest for 10 minutes before slicing. Serve the steak with steamed veggies, over a salad, or in a taco.

Nutrition

Calories: 312kcal | Carbohydrates: 10g | Protein: 25g | Fat: 19g | Saturated Fat: 4g | Cholesterol: 68mg | Sodium: 64mg | Potassium: 432mg | Fiber: 1g | Sugar: 6g | Vitamin A: 296IU | Vitamin C: 13mg | Calcium: 41mg | Iron: 2mg

Air Fryer Ribeye Steak (Frozen + Fresh)

Prep Time: 5 Minutes

Cook Time: 10 Minutes

Additional Time: 30 Minutes

Total Time: 45 Minutes

Ingredients

- 8-ounce ribeye steak, about 1-inch thick
- 1 tablespoon McCormick Montreal Steak Seasoning

Instructions

Remove the ribeye steak from the fridge and season with the Montreal Steak seasoning. Let steak rest for about 20 minutes to come to room temperature (to get a more tender juicy steak).

Preheat your air fryer to 400 degrees.

Place the ribeye steak in the air fryer and cook for 10-12 minutes, until it reaches 130-135 degrees for medium-rare. Cook for an additional 5 minutes for medium-well.

Remove the steak from the air fryer and let rest at least 5 minutes before cutting to keep the juices inside the steak then enjoy!

Nutrition Information

Total Fat: 22g| Saturated Fat: 10g| Trans Fat: 0g| Unsaturated Fat: 12g| Cholesterol: 88mg| Sodium: 789mg| Carbohydrates: 2g| Fiber: 1g| Sugar: 0g| Protein: 29g

Air Fryer Beef Chips

Prep Time: 1 minute

Cook Time: 1 hour

Cooling Time: 5 minutes

Total Time: 1 hour 6 minutes

Servings: 2

Ingredients

- 1/2 lb Thinly Sliced Beef we recommend leaner cuts like sirloin 1/4 tsp Salt
- 1/4 tsp Black Pepper
- 1/4 tsp Garlic Powder

Instructions

Gather all the ingredients.

In a small mixing bowl, combine salt, black pepper, garlic powder and mix well to create the seasoning.

Lay the beef slices flat and sprinkle seasoning on both sides.

Transfer beef into the air fryer tray single stacked (very important each slice is single stacked, otherwise they will not get crispy) and air fry for 45-60 minutes at 200F. Once done, let beef slices cool for 5 minutes before enjoying. Note - the time is going to vary greatly depending on thickness.

Nutrition Information

Calories: 290kcal | Carbohydrates: 1g | Protein: 20g | Fat: 23g | Saturated Fat: 9g | Cholesterol: 81mg | Sodium: 367mg | Potassium: 306mg | Sugar: 1g | Calcium: 20mg | Iron: 2mg

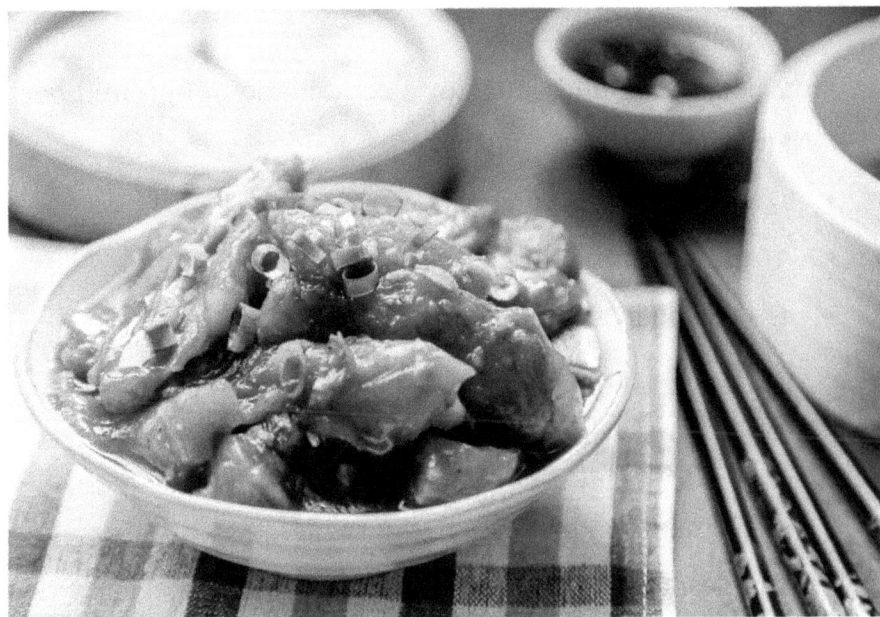

Best Air Fryer Meatloaf With Tangy Sauce | Makes Two

Prep Time: 9 Mins

Cook Time: 20 Mins

Resting Time: 5 Mins

Total Time: 34 Mins

Ingredients

- 1 large egg
- 2 pounds ground chuck or a combination of ground beef and venison or ground sirloin
- 1/2 cup quick-cooking oats
- 3/4 teaspoon salt or garlic salt
- 1/4 teaspoon ground black pepper

Tangy sauce

- 3/4 cup ketchup
- 2   tablespoons light brown sugar
- 1 tablespoon apple cider vinegar or white vinegar or rice vinegar

- 1 teaspoon worcestershire sauce or soy sauce or liquid amino liquid aminos are gluten-free

Instructions

To save washing another bowl, start by beating the egg in a large bowl with a fork.

Break up the ground meat in the bowl. There's no getting around using your hands here. I usually use a pair of nylon/rubber gloves simply for easy cleanup. Gloves may be a luxury this day, though.

Add quick-cooking oats, salt, and pepper.

With your hands, gently mix in the egg, oats, salt, and pepper with the ground meat. Overworking the meat will make it tough. Under mixing may leave patches of oats or eggs not evenly incorporated.

Shape the mixture into 2 free-form loaves, roughly 3 x 5.5 inches. The size will depend on what will fit into your air fryer. (For conventional oven method, see the size in recipe notes) Carefully place the loaves side by side in the preheated air fryer basket or tray.

Air fry or Roast for about 19 minutes or until meatloaves are done in the middle-firm when pressed in the middle of temperature on an instant-read thermometer reads 155°.

It's a good idea to check at 17 minutes to make sure they aren't getting too brown. All air fryers are not alike.

Prepare Tangy Sauce and Spread on Meatloaf

Stir or whisk together ketchup, brown sugar, vinegar, and Worcestershire sauce.

When meat waves are 155° or no pink shows in the center, evenly spread the Tangy Sauce over both meatloaves. Cook an additional 1 minute on Air Fry to set the sauce.

Remove the meatloaves with silicone coated tongs if the air fryer basket is coated with a nonstick surface. Let the meatloaf stand on a cutting board or plate 5 minutes before slicing.

Nutritional Value

Calories: 572kcal | Carbohydrates: 1g | Protein: 46g | Fat: 43g | Saturated Fat: 22g | Cholesterol: 168mg

| Sodium: 219mg | Potassium: 606mg | Sugar: 1g | Vitamin A: 355IU | Calcium: 16mg | Iron: 4mg

Air Fryer Asian Beef & Veggies

Prep Time: 10 minutes

Cook Time: 8 minutes

Total Time: 18 minutes

Servings: 4 people

Ingredients

- 1 lb sirloin steak cut into strips
- 2 tablespoons cornstarch (or arrowroot powder)
- 1/2 medium yellow onion, sliced
- 1 medium red pepper, sliced into strips
- 3 cloves garlic, minced
- 2 tablespoons grated ginger do not sub dry ground ginger
- 1/4 teaspoon red chili flakes
- 1/2 cup low sodium soy sauce
- 1/4 cup rice vinegar
- 1 tsp sesame oil
- 1/3 cup brown sugar
- 1 teaspoon chinese 5 spice optional
- 1/4 cup water

Instructions

For Freezer Prep

Add all ingredients to a gallon-sized zip bag. Ensure all of the ingredients are combined. Label and freeze for up to 4 months.

To Cook

Thaw zip bag in the fridge overnight.

Using tongs, remove the steak and veggies, and transfer to the Air Fryer. Discard the marinade.

Set the Air Fryer to 400F and the timer to 8 minutes. I like to shake the basket halfway through, but I don't think it is necessary.

Serve with rice, and garnish with sesame seeds and scallions.

Nutrition

Calories: 289kcal | Carbohydrates: 27g | Protein: 31g | Fat: 7g | Fiber: 1g | Sugar: 19g

Kofta Kebabs

Prep Time: 45 mins

Cook Time: 5 mins

Additional Time: 30 mins

Total Time: 1 hr 20 mins

Servings: 28

Ingredient

- 4 cloves garlic, minced
- 1 teaspoon kosher salt
- 1 pound ground lamb
- 3 tablespoons grated onion
- 3 tablespoons chopped fresh parsley
- 1 tablespoon ground coriander
- 1 teaspoon ground cumin
- ½ tablespoon ground cinnamon
- ½ teaspoon ground allspice
- ¼ teaspoon cayenne pepper
- ¼ teaspoon ground ginger
- ¼ teaspoon ground black pepper
- 28 bamboo skewers, soaked in water for 30 minutes

Instructions

Mash the garlic into a paste with the salt using a mortar and pestle or the flat side of a chef's knife on your cutting board. Mix the garlic into the lamb along with the onion, parsley, coriander, cumin, cinnamon, allspice, cayenne pepper, ginger, and pepper in a mixing bowl until well blended. Form the mixture into 28 balls. Form each ball around the tip of a skewer, flattening into a 2-inch oval; repeat with the remaining skewers. Place the kebabs onto a baking sheet, cover, and refrigerate for at least 30 minutes or up to 12 hours.

Preheat an outdoor grill for medium heat, and lightly oil grate.

Cook the skewers on the preheated grill, turning occasionally, until the lamb has cooked to your desired degree of doneness, about 6 minutes for medium.

Nutrition Facts

Calories: 35; Protein 2.9g; Carbohydrates 0.6g; Fat 2.3g; Cholesterol 10.8mg; Sodium 78.2mg.

Simple Grilled Lamb Chops

Prep Time: 10 mins

Cook Time: 6 mins

Additional Time: 2 hrs

Total Time: 2 hrs 16 mins

Servings: 6

Ingredient

- ¼ cup distilled white vinegar
- 2 teaspoons salt
- ½ teaspoon black pepper
- 1 tablespoon minced garlic
- 1 onion, thinly sliced
- 2 tablespoons olive oil
- 2 pounds lamb chops

Instructions

Mix together the vinegar, salt, pepper, garlic, onion, and olive oil in a large resealable bag until the salt has dissolved. Add lamb, toss until coated, and marinate in the refrigerator for 2 hours.

Preheat an outdoor grill for medium-high heat.

Remove lamb from the marinade and leave any onions on that stick to the meat. Discard any remaining marinade. Wrap the exposed ends of the bones with aluminum foil to keep them from burning. Grill to desired doneness, about 3 minutes per side for medium. The chops may also be broiled in the oven for about 5 minutes per side for medium.

Nutrition Facts

Calories: 519; Protein 25g; Carbohydrates 2.3g; Fat 44.8g; Cholesterol 112mg; Sodium 861mg.

Roast Leg Of Lamb

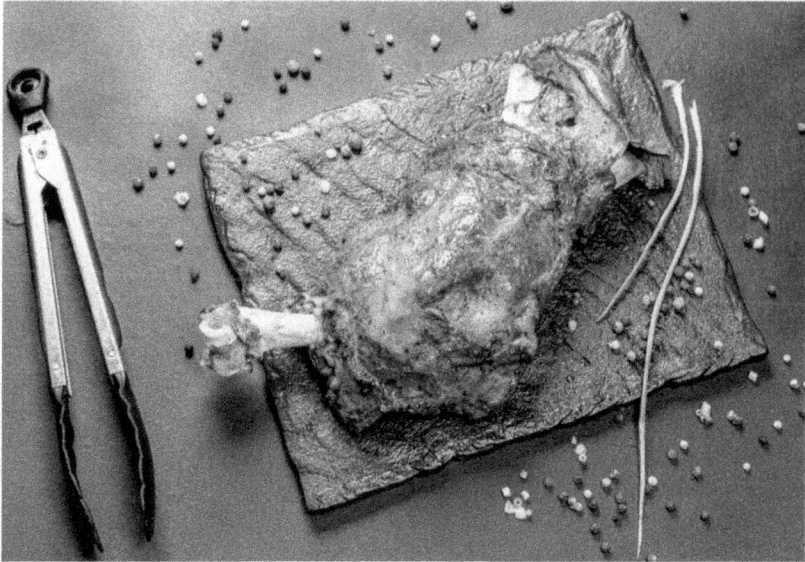

Prep Time: 15 mins

Cook Time: 1 hr 45 mins

Additional Time: 10 mins

Total Time: 2 hrs 10 mins

Servings: 12

Ingredient

4 cloves garlic, sliced

2 tablespoons fresh rosemary

Salt to taste

Ground black pepper to taste

5 pounds leg of lamb

Instructions

Preheat oven to 350 degrees F (175 degrees C).

Cut slits in the top of the leg of lamb every 3 to 4 inches, deep enough to push slices of garlic down into the meat. Salt and pepper generously all over the top of the lamb, place several sprigs of fresh rosemary under and on top of the lamb. Place lamb on roasting pan.

Roast in the preheated oven until the lamb is cooked to your desired doneness, about 1 3/4 to 2 hours. Do not overcook the lamb, the flavor is best if the meat is still slightly pink. Let rest at least 10 minutes before carving.

Nutrition Facts

Calories: 382; Protein 35.8g; Carbohydrates 0.4g; Fat 25.3g; Cholesterol 136.1mg; Sodium 136.3mg.

Roasted Lamb Breast

Prep Time: 30 mins

Cook Time: 2 hrs 25 mins

Total Time: 2 hrs 55 mins

Servings: 4

Ingredient

- 2 tablespoons olive oil
- 2 teaspoons salt
- 2 teaspoons ground cumin
- 1 teaspoon freshly ground black pepper
- 1 teaspoon dried Italian herb seasoning
- 1 teaspoon ground cinnamon
- 1 teaspoon ground coriander
- 1 teaspoon paprika
- 4 pounds lamb breast, separated into two pieces
- ½ cup chopped Italian flat-leaf parsley
- ⅓ cup white wine vinegar, more as needed
- 1 lemon, juiced
- 2 cloves garlic, crushed
- 1 teaspoon honey

- ½ teaspoon red pepper flakes
- 1 pinch salt

Instructions

Preheat oven to 300 degrees F (150 degrees C).

Combine chopped parsley, vinegar, fresh lemon juice, garlic, honey, red pepper flakes, and salt in a large bowl. Mix well and set aside.

Whisk olive oil, salt, cumin, black pepper, dried Italian herbs, cinnamon, coriander, and paprika in a large bowl until combined.

Coat each lamb breast in the olive oil and spice mixture and transfer to a roasting pan, fat side up. Tightly cover the roasting pan with aluminum foil and bake in the preheated oven until the meat is tender when pierced with a fork, about 2 hours.

Remove lamb from the oven and cut into four pieces. Increase oven temperature to 450 degrees F (230 degrees C).

Line a baking sheet with aluminum foil and place lamb pieces on it. Brush the tops of each piece with fat drippings from the roasting pan.

Bake lamb until meat is browned and edges are crispy about 20 minutes.

Increase the oven's broiler to high and brown lamb for 4 minutes. Remove from oven. Serve lamb topped with parsley and vinegar sauce.

Nutrition Facts

Calories: 622; Protein 46.2g; Carbohydrates 7.7g; Fat 45.3g; Cholesterol 180.4mg; Sodium 1301.6mg.

Moroccan Lamb Stew With Apricots

Prep Time: 30 mins

Cook Time: 1 hr 55 mins

Total Time: 2 hrs 25 mins

Servings: 4

Ingredient

- 2 pounds boneless leg of lamb, cut into 1-inch cubes
- 2 teaspoons ground coriander
- 1 teaspoon ground cumin
- 1 teaspoon sweet paprika
- ½ teaspoon cayenne pepper
- ½ teaspoon ground cardamom
- ½ teaspoon ground turmeric
- 2 teaspoons kosher salt
- 2 tablespoons olive oil
- 2 cups finely chopped onion
- 4 cloves garlic, minced
- 1 tablespoon minced fresh ginger root
- 2 (3 inches) cinnamon sticks

- 2 cups low-sodium chicken stock
- 1 cup dried apricots, halved
- 2 (3 inches) orange peel strips
- 1 tablespoon honey
- ¼ cup chopped fresh cilantro
- ¼ cup toasted pine nuts

Instructions

Combine lamb, coriander, cumin, paprika, cayenne, cardamom, turmeric, and salt in a large bowl; toss together until lamb is evenly coated.

Heat oil in a large Dutch oven or tagine over medium heat. Add onions; cook, stirring occasionally until soft and translucent, about 5 minutes. Stir in garlic, ginger, and cinnamon; cook, stirring frequently, until fragrant, about 1 minute. Add seasoned lamb; cook, stirring fre🢂uently until light brown, being careful not to caramelize, about 2 minutes. Add chicken stock and bring to a gentle boil over medium heat. Reduce heat to low and simmer, covered, until the lamb is just tender, about 1 hour and 15 minutes.

Stir in apricots, orange peels, and honey; continue to simmer over low heat, uncovered, until the liquid has thickened slightly and lamb is fork-tender, about 30 minutes. Remove from the heat, discard cinnamon sticks and orange peels.

Divide evenly among 4 bowls. Garnish each bowl with a tablespoon each of cilantro and pine nuts.

Nutrition Facts

Calories: 553; Protein 44.5g; Carbohydrates 40.9g; Fat 24.8g; Cholesterol 125.5mg; Sodium 1129.7mg.

Slow Cooker Lamb Chops

Prep Time: 15 mins

Cook Time: 4 hrs 30 mins

Additional Time: 5 mins

Total Time: 4 hrs 50 mins

Servings: 6

Ingredient

- ½ cup red wine
- ½ sweet onion, roughly chopped
- 3 tablespoons honey
- 2 tablespoons Dijon mustard
- 2 tablespoons lemon juice
- 4 garlic cloves, minced
- 1 tablespoon ground thyme
- tablespoon dried rosemary
- 2 teaspoons ground basil
- 1 teaspoon salt
- 1 teaspoon coarse ground black pepper
- ¼ cup tapioca starch
- 1 ½ pound sirloin lamb chops, room temperature

Instructions

Combine red wine and onion in a slow cooker.

Whisk honey, mustard, lemon juice, garlic, thyme, rosemary, basil, salt, and pepper together in a small bowl until well blended. Add tapioca starch and whisk until well combined. Let sit until the mixture is thickened, at least 5 minutes.

Dip lamb chops in the mustard mixture and massage until fully coated.

Place chops in a single layer over the red wine and onion mixture in the slow cooker. Pour the remaining mustard mixture on top.

Cover slow cooker and cook on Low until an instant-read thermometer inserted into the center of a chop reads at least 130 degrees F (54 degrees C), about 4 1/2 hours.

Nutrition Facts

Calories: 209; Protein 13g; Carbohydrates 18.5g; Fat 7.7g; Cholesterol 43.6mg; Sodium 550.5mg.

Grilled Leg Of Lamb Steaks

Prep Time: 10 mins

Cook Time: 10 mins

Additional Time: 30 mins

Total: 50 mins

Servings: 4

Ingredient

4 bone-in lamb steaks

¼ cup olive oil

4 large cloves garlic, minced

1 tablespoon chopped fresh rosemary

Salt and ground black pepper to taste

Instructions

Place lamb steaks in a single layer in a shallow dish. Cover with olive oil, garlic, rosemary, salt, and pepper. Flip steaks to coat both sides. Let sit until steaks absorb flavors, about 30 minutes.

Preheat an outdoor grill for high heat and lightly oil the grate. Cook steaks until browned on the outside and slightly pink in the center, about 5 minutes per side for medium. An instant-read thermometer inserted into the center should read at least 140 degrees F (60 degrees C).

Nutrition Facts

Calories: 327; Protein 29.6g; Carbohydrates 1.7g; Fat 21.9g; Cholesterol 92.9mg; Sodium 112.1mg.

Easy Meatloaf

Prep Time: 10 mins

Cook Time: 1 hr

Total Time: 1 hr 10 mins

Servings: 8

Ingredient

- 1 ½ pounds ground beef
- 1 egg
- 1 onion, chopped
- 1 cup milk
- 1 cup dried bread crumbs
- Salt and pepper to taste
- 2 tablespoons brown sugar
- 2 tablespoons prepared mustard
- ⅓ cup ketchup

Instructions

Preheat oven to 350 degrees F (175 degrees C).

In a large bowl, combine the beef, egg, onion, milk, and bread OR cracker crumbs. Season with salt and pepper to taste and place in a lightly greased 9x5-inch loaf pan, or form into a loaf and place in a lightly greased 9x13-inch baking dish.

In a separate small bowl, combine the brown sugar, mustard, and ketchup. Mix well and pour over the meatloaf.

Bake at 350 degrees F (175 degrees C) for 1 hour.

Nutrition Facts

Calories: 372; Protein 18.2g; Carbohydrates 18.5g; Fat 24.7g; Cholesterol 98mg; Sodium 334.6mg.

Classic Meatloaf

Prep: 30 mins

Cook: 45 mins

Total: 1 hr 15 mins

Servings: 10

Meatloaf Ingredients:

- 1 carrot, coarsely chopped
- 1 rib celery, coarsely chopped
- ½ onion, coarsely chopped
- ½ red bell pepper, coarsely chopped
- 4 white mushrooms, coarsely chopped
- 3 cloves garlic, coarsely chopped
- 2 ½ pounds ground chuck
- 1 tablespoon Worcestershire sauce
- 1 egg, beaten
- 1 teaspoon dried Italian herbs
- 2 teaspoons salt
- 1 teaspoon ground black pepper
- ½ teaspoon cayenne pepper
- 1 cup plain bread crumbs

- 1 teaspoon olive oil

Glaze Ingredients:

- 2 tablespoons brown sugar
- 2 tablespoons ketchup
- 2 tablespoons dijon mustard
- Hot pepper sauce to taste

Instructions

Preheat the oven to 325 degrees F.

Place the carrot, celery, onion, red bell pepper, mushrooms, and garlic in a food processor, and pulse until very finely chopped, almost to a puree. Place the minced vegetables into a large mixing bowl, and mix in ground chuck, Worcestershire sauce, and egg. Add Italian herbs, salt, black pepper, and cayenne pepper. Mix gently with a wooden spoon to incorporate vegetables and egg into the meat. Pour in bread crumbs. With your hand, gently mix in the crumbs with your fingertips just until combined, about 1 minute.

Form the meatloaf into a ball. Pour olive oil into a baking dish and place the ball of meat into the dish. Shape the ball into a loaf, about 4 inches high by 6 inches across.

Bake in the preheated oven just until the meatloaf is hot, about 15 minutes.

Meanwhile, in a small bowl, mix together brown sugar, ketchup, Dijon mustard, and hot sauce. Stir until the brown sugar has dissolved.

Remove the meatloaf from the oven. With the back of a spoon, smooth the glaze onto the top of the meatloaf, then pull a little bit of glaze down the sides of the meatloaf with the back of the spoon.

Return meatloaf to the oven, and bake until the loaf is no longer pink inside and the glaze has baked onto the loaf, 30 to 40 more minutes. An instant-read thermometer inserted into the thickest part of the loaf should read at least 160 degrees F (70 degrees C). Cooking time will depend on the shape and thickness of the meatloaf.

Nutrition Facts

Calories: 284; Protein 21.6g; Carbohydrates 14.8g; Fat 14.9g; Cholesterol 85.3mg; Sodium 755.4mg.

Salisbury Steak

Prep Time: 20 mins

Cook Time: 20 mins

Total Time: 40 mins

Servings: 6

Ingredient

- 1 (10.5 ounces) can condense French onion soup
- 1 ½ pounds ground beef
- ½ cup dry bread crumbs
- 1 egg
- ¼ teaspoon salt
- ⅛ teaspoon ground black pepper
- 1 tablespoon all-purpose flour
- ¼ cup ketchup
- ¼ cup water
- 1 tablespoon Worcestershire sauce
- ½ teaspoon mustard powder

Instructions

In a large bowl, mix together 1/3 cup condensed French onion soup with ground beef, bread crumbs, egg, salt, and black pepper. Shape into 6 oval patties.

In a large skillet over medium-high heat, brown both sides of patties. Pour off excess fat.

In a small bowl, blend flour and remaining soup until smooth. Mix in ketchup, water, Worcestershire sauce, and mustard powder. Pour over meat in skillet. Cover, and cook for 20 minutes, stirring occasionally.

Nutrition Facts

Calories: 440; Protein 23g; Carbohydrates 14.1g; Fat 32.3g; Cholesterol 127.5mg; Sodium 818.3mg.

Marinated Air Fryer Vegetables

Prep Time: 10 minutes

Cook Time: 15 minutes

Marinading time: 20 minutes

Total Time: 25 minutes

Servings: 4 servings

Ingredients

Vegetables

- 2 green zucchini cut into ½ inch pieces
- 1 yellow squash cut into ½ inch pieces
- 4 oz button mushrooms cut in half
- 1 red onion cut into ½ inch pieces
- 1 red bell pepper cut into ½ inch pieces Marinade
- 4 Tbsp Olive Oil
- 2 Tbsp Balsamic Vinegar
- 1 Tbsp Honey
- 1 ½ tsp salt
- ½ tsp dried thyme
- ½ tsp dried oregano
- ¼ tsp garlic powder

- A few drops of liquid smoke optional
- Salt to taste

Instructions

Place marinade ingredients in a large bowl and whisk until combined. Place chopped vegetables in a bowl and stir until all vegetables are fully covered.

Allow vegetables to marinate for 20-30 minutes.

Place marinated vegetables in an air fryer basket and cook at 400 degrees Fahrenheit for 15-18 minutes, stirring every 5 minutes, until tender. Salt to taste.

Nutrition

Calories: 200kcal | Carbohydrates: 16g | Protein: 3g | Fat: 15g | Saturated Fat: 2g | Sodium: 890mg | Potassium: 586mg | Fiber: 3g | Sugar: 12g | Vitamin A: 1225IU | Vitamin C: 67mg | Calcium: 34mg | Iron: 1mg

Airfried Vegetables

Prep time: 10 min

Cook time: 20 min

Total time: 30 min

Serves: 4

Ingredients

- 1 lb / 0.5kg of vegetables (broccoli, brussels sprouts, carrots, cauliflower, parsnips, potatoes, sweet potatoes, zucchini will all work), chopped evenly
- 1 Tbsp / 30 mL of cooking oil
- Some salt and pepper

Instructions

Prep

Preheat air fryer for about 5 minutes at 360F / 182C degrees.

Evenly chop veggies and toss with oil and some salt and pepper. If making potato or sweet potato fries, soak them in water for ~30 minutes to draw out excess starch for crispier results, and then pat dry thoroughly with paper towels before tossing with oil.

Make

Transfer veggies into frying compartment and fry for 15 to 20 minutes, stirring veggies every 5 to 8 minutes or so. Some veggies might need longer and some will need less – just use your judgment when you open the compartment to stir the veggies. You want the outside to be golden and crispy and the inside to be tender.

Enjoy or toss with your favorite dipping sauce when done! If you need sauce ideas, check out 5 of our favorites.

Nutrition Information

Calories: 172 Total Fat: 11g Saturated Fat: 2g

Unsaturated Fat: 9g Sodium: 577mg Carbohydrates: 16g Fiber: 6g

Sugar: 4g Protein: 6g

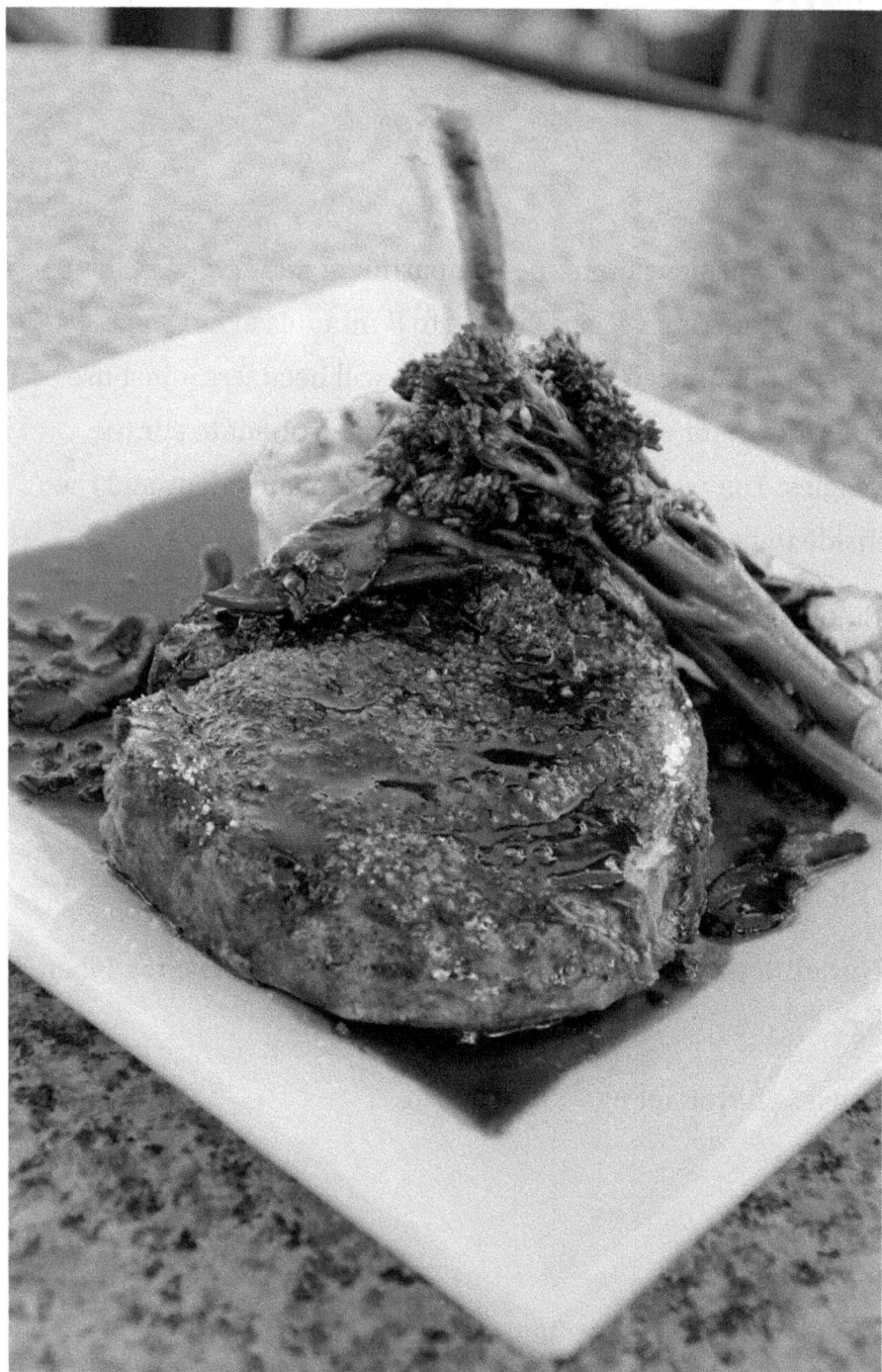

www.ingramcontent.com/pod-product-compliance
Lightning Source LLC
Chambersburg PA
CBHW050748030426
42336CB00012B/1720